Clary Sage Essential Oils

Benefits, Properties, Applications, Studies & Recipes

by Ann Sullivan

Published in USA by:

Ann Sullivan
217 N. Seacrest Blvd #9
Boynton Beach
FL 33425

© Copyright 2015

ISBN-13: ISBN-13: 978-1544754727
ISBN-10: ISBN-10: 1544754728

Table of Contents

Introduction

What are essential oils and how might they be used for therapeutic purposes?

Essential oils are ultra-potent oils extracted from plants and flowers that have been utilized in medicine for centuries. Presently, they are most commonly used to supplement pharmaceutical medication, but they can also be an effective alternative to pharmaceuticals in the event that there is no access to them. Before dismissing essential oils as a means to support the body's natural defenses against injury and illness, take a look at the historical evidence of the oils' therapeutic competence in practice. The average age-old medical text will demonstrate that essential oils, herbs, and plenty of other natural ingredients have, for thousands of years, successfully enhanced immune function to meet and defeat any number of ailments and injuries. Though traditional medicine is considered "alternative" now, it was once the gold standard. Perhaps it still should be, as these natural age-tested remedies can fortify the body's defenses against everything from simple maladies, like headaches, cuts, and bruises to serious diseases, like cancer.

Essential oils are deemed "essential," because the oils are composed of the "essence" of the plant. The difference between essential oils and other oils – like olive oil or vegetable oil, for instance – is that essential oils have high volatility and reduced fixation, which results in faster evaporation, enabling their popular use in aromatherapy. Even at high temperatures, olive and vegetable oils do not evaporate.

Essential oils are especially necessary when it comes to a major natural or man-made disaster or potential viral outbreak. In these dire situations, people may not have quick access to their standard pharmaceutical supply; so essential oils, along with other alternative medicines, will be the go-to wellness aids in the case of social collapse, viral outbreak, or devastating natural disaster. When medical access is unavailable, alternatives to our modern-day standard are the only chance we have to keep pathogens at bay.

Most people do not realize that they already use essential oils every day. They are in perfumes, shampoos, soaps, and ointments; they are even used in furniture polish. Why are they found in so many aromatic products? Well, because essential oils are super concentrated aromatic liquids, so their scent is remarkably strong. Let us put this into perspective: to steam tea, use a few leaves of peppermint or juniper; to produce a single ounce of essential oil, five whole *pounds* of peppermint or juniper leaves are required. Some sources claim that to produce twelve pounds of essential oil would necessitate an acre of peppermint, juniper, or any other oil being produced en masse. Unlike vegetable oil, you do not often find concentrated therapeutic-grade essential oils sold in bulk; instead the oils are often sold in easily carried small, dark bottles, perfect for the GOOD bag (Get Out Of Dodge). That is exactly what this book is aiming to help people plan for – getting out of dodge with the most vital of essential oils intact, in particular a good supply of Clary Sage essential oil.

Why Clary Sage, you ask? Well, in order to get quickly up to speed on this most essential of oils, below we have provided a condensed synopsis of Clary Sage, after which we will outline in greater detail the oil's history, properties, and common therapeutic uses, so that you – the consumer – might have a better understanding of the oil's benefits and applications. We have even provided supportive remedies for pure Clary Sage, as well as blended recipes that incorporate the valuable oil. Chapter 3 will further detail past scientific research on Clary Sage essential oil.

Now, let's get down to it.

Essential Oil 101: The Basics of Clary Sage

Summary: Clary Sage, or Salvia sclarea, is a very female-friendly oil, having been used for centuries in supporting a great number of women's issues, from PMS to labor pains. However, not only does it aid women's hormonal imbalances, the sclareol within balances male hormones as well. Scareol is a diterpene alcohol, whose chemical composition is similar to that of the hormones within the human body. Thus, it helps stimulate the production of hormones, providing the body hormonal balance, particularly estrogen balance.

Description: Clary Sage oil is commonly extracted through steam distillation. The flowers, buds, or leaves are most often used. The oil is light gold in color, medium thin in consistency, and has a somewhat strong earthy and herb-like scent.

Uses: Beyond those applications previously mentioned, additional uses for Clary Sage essential oil include supporting PMS and other menstrual issues, pre-menopause, hormonal imbalance, hemorrhoids, bronchitis, impotence, circulatory issues, high cholesterol, insomnia, flatulence, amenorrhea, asthma, sore throat, coughing, kidney disorders, hair loss and labor pains. When it comes to mood and emotion, Clary Sage can help relieve stress, anxiety, fear, loneliness, fatigue and exhaustion.

Properties: Antispasmodic, anticonvulsive, antifungal, antidepressant, antiseptic, antibacterial, sedative, euphoric, carminative, aphrodisiac, astringent, digestive, emmenagogue, nervine, stomachic, hypotensive, tonic, and uterine.

Application: Dilute 1:1 with a carrier oil. Apply topically, inhale directly, diffuse or use as a dietary supplement.

Safety Precautions: Clary Sage has been approved by the FDA for internal consumption and can be used as a dietary supplement. Do not use when drinking alcohol as Clary Sage has a narcotic effect. Those who have breast cancer should avoid Clary Sage as it has an estrogen-like effect.

Fun facts: Clary Sage's botanical name has Latin roots, with clary derived from the Latin word for "clear" ("clarus") and salvia derived from the Latin word for "to heal or save" ("salvere").

These Latin roots may also have inspired Clary Sage's medieval nickname "Clear Eyes," which it was called for its use in healing eye conditions.

Chapter 1:
Benefits of Clary Sage Essential Oil

Clary Sage essential oil offers a number of therapeutic benefits; but you may be wondering what these benefits are. In this chapter, we'll take a closer look at the history of Clary Sage and its many uses.

Cultivation of Clary Sage

Clary Sage is often a biennial plant but at times can be a short-term perennial when of the genus Salvia. As a biennial its germination period lasts from 12 - 15 days. When the plant is cultivated it grows best in 70° Fahrenheit soil in a humid climate with full direct sunlight. Clary Sage can tolerate dry conditions but the soil must be fertile and well drained. Planted 2-3 feet apart Clary Sage grows up to 4 feet tall, with thick furry stems and large leaves, about a foot long at the base and half a foot at higher points on the plant. Lilac, pink, white, or mauve flowers, about 1-inch-wide, also grow on the plant, which sows itself. Those seedlings planted in the spring will flower during the next season. Salvia sclarea is native to the northern Mediterranean, central Asia, and northern Africa regions, and its long history as a therapeutic herb has made it a commonly cultivated plant.

A History of Clary Sage

Clary Sage is said to have originated either in central and southwest Europe or in Syria where it continues to flourish. The essential oil of Clary Sage was mentioned by Dioscorides and Pliny the Elder in the 1st century BC, and Theophrastus during the 4th century BC, three Greek physicians and botanists. The oil also served as a fixer in perfumery and cosmetics, particularly in Russia and France. It was even used in shampoos, creams, and ointments, as it helped stimulate sebum production.

Clary Sage is a close relative of cooking sage and in fact can also be used for cooking; wild or cultivated. However, Clary Sage is now most often cultivated in order to extract its essential oils, as the oil's components have been shown to support the hypothalamus, the part of the brain that responds to fear, paranoia, and anxiety, thus helping to relieve psychological issues. True to its name, Clary Sage is also said to promote clarity of thought and calm, making it a common recommendation when it comes to menstrual issues, like PMS, insomnia, and cramping.

The mucilaginous coat of the plant's seeds has prompted its use in eye care. When a seed is placed in the eye, whatever foreign object is irritating the eye will adhere to the seed and become more easy to remove. The practice is noted by Nicholas Culpeper, a 17th century herbalist. The seed of Clary Sage has long been said to clear up red eyes and eye infections, or conditions as well, prompting its medieval nickname "clear eyes." In fact, Clary Sage derived its scientific name from the plant's reputation for clearing up the eyes as well. The Latin word "sclarea," which is also the species' name, comes from "clarus," meaning "clear." The plant's genus, "salvia," means "to save." This is because the sage family of plants was believed to be a natural savior since ancient times.

Culpeper also suggested the use of Clary Sage as an aphrodisiac and a kidney supporter. The oil also stimulates estrogen production and so should be avoided by women who are pregnant.

Old Clary Sage leaves have a bitter taste, but the young leaves are sometimes eaten raw or used to season dishes. The plant's flowers as well can be used in salads. Moreover, Clary Sage has traditionally been a flavoring for wine, ale, vermouth, and various liqueurs. When combined with other flowering blossoms and herbs, Clary Sage can provide a muscatel flavor to wine.

Chemical Components

In order to generate the essential oil from Clary Sage, the flowers, buds, and leaves must be steam distilled. This results in the oil's key chemical components, which are primarily sclareol, linalyl acetate, linalool, caryophyllene, geraniol, a-terpineol, neryl acetate, and germacrene D.

Main Properties of Clary Sage Essential Oil

Along with the properties previously mentioned in the introduction, Clary Sage oil possesses antispasmodic, anticonvulsive, antifungal, antidepressant, antiseptic, antibacterial, sedative, euphoric, carminative, aphrodisiac, astringent, digestive, emmenagogue, nervine, stomachic, hypotensive, tonic, and uterine properties. With such a versatile range Clary Sage is well equipped to fight off any pathogen in the body's path.

Clary Sage as mentioned is composed of sclareol, linalyl acetate, linalool, caryophyllene, geraniol, a-terpineol, neryl acetate, and germacrene D. These components are what instill the enormously beneficial properties within Clary Sage essential oil. We will outline these properties below.

Antioxidant

Anything high in antioxidants – whether fruit, beans, or essential oils – is a powerful advocate for the body. Antioxidants both protect against free radicals and repair their damage. What are free radicals? Free radicals are destructive chemicals that invade the body produced by substances both inside and out. Some free radicals (or oxidants) form through normal bodily reactions, like inflammation, metabolism, and aerobic respiration. Other free radicals form outside the body but enter it due to exposure. These include harmful pollutants, toxins, smoking, alcohol, X-rays, and UV rays, to name a few. Although our bodies produce their own antioxidants these often become damaged as we grow older; introducing antioxidants into our bodies allows these nutrients and enzymes to assist in chemical reactions which destroy the oxidants or free radicals. Clary Sage essential oil is a moderate antioxidant aiming to detox the body of free radicals that lead to disease.

Antispasmodic

The antispasmodic properties of Clary Sage oil make it beneficial to such surgical processes as colonoscopy, gastroscopy, and intra-luminally-applied double-contrast barium enema.

Antifungal

While bacteria and viruses are plenty evil, fungi commonly lead to the deadliest infections, whether external or internal. The ears, throat, and nose are the most likely to become infected by fungi, the infections of which can be both excruciating and unsightly. If left untreated fungal infections can kill, as they may spread to the brain. Clary Sage essential oil protects against these infections and more and is particularly effective against skin infections.

Antidepressant

When it comes to psychological issues the uplifting scent of Clary Sage combats negative thoughts and thereby depression.

Antiseptic

The antiseptic and disinfectant properties of Clary Sage essential oil can be reaped topically, applied directly to wounds, or even through burning; the smoke from the oil may help destroy airborne germs. Internal use will help keep the wounds from becoming infections, while external use will support the body's natural function in inhibiting tetanus.

Antibacterial

Clary Sage's antibacterial properties make it a powerful protectant against diseases produced by bacteria, such as oral, digestive and urinary tract bacterial infection. What's great is that, unlike some prescription drugs, Clary Sage has no ill effects on body wellness, or on the healthy natural flora that exists within the stomach and intestines.

Sedative

As a sedative, Clary Sage sedates and calms by reducing anxiety, excitement or irritability. Though sedatives, alone, do not alleviate pain, they do calm the patient, making them less stressed and more compliant.

Carminative

By supporting the reduction of excess gas buildup and/or removal of gas from the intestines, Clary Sage essential oil provides relief from abdominal pain, excess sweating, and uncomfortable indigestion.

Aphrodisiac

As an aphrodisiac, Clary Sage can help stimulate sexual arousal, thereby overriding impotence, frigidity, low libido, and erectile dysfunction.

Astringent

For those who do not know what an astringent is, it is a chemical compound that shrinks body tissues, which means it can aid skin issues and irritations, everything from acne to insect bites. The astringent property of Clary Sage essential oil benefits everything from skin to hair to gums to muscles to intestines. As an astringent, Clary Sage is an anti-agent, combating muscle loss through the ability to strengthen. This astringent and coagulant properties also mean that diarrhea can be relieved through use of Clary Sage essential oil, as well as wound and cut bleeding.

Digestive

By boosting the production of absorptive enzymes, the digestibility of nutrients, and the secretion of digestive juices, Clary Sage essential oil aids the digestive tract significantly, which can make a great impact on the body's overall wellness by increasing those nutrients absorbed from food.

Emmenagogue

No need to look this one up. An emmenagogue is a menstrual stimulant for those with irregular menses. Clary Sage regulates hormones which means that this emmenagogue can also delay and/or reduce the symptoms of menopause, which include hormonal and mood imbalance, nausea, pain, headache, and fatigue..

Stomachic

As a stomachic, Clary Sage improves stomach function, boosts appetite, and helps to tone the stomach. The oil helps control the stomach's bile, acid, and gastric liquids.

Uterine

Clary Sage essential oil helps regulate the menstrual cycle, as well as gynecological conditions. Furthermore, Clary Sage can protect against uterine cancer by regulating estrogen production, thereby decreasing the risk of uterine cyst and tumor formation after menopause.

Tonic

Clary Sage essential oil benefits each of the body's systems, whether nervous, digestive, respiratory, or excretory, making it an unbeatable general tonic. The oil also supports the immune system by helping the body absorb nutrients.

Nervine

As a nervine, Clary Sage helps calm nervous convulsions and nervous conditions, like anxiety, hysteria, and vertigo.

Hypotensive

By supporting the relaxation of veins and arteries Clary Sage effectively reduces blood pressure. This boosts circulation and oxygenation to the organ systems and muscles, improving their function, as well as your metabolism, while also reducing the body's vulnerability to such risks as stroke, heart attack, brain hemorrhaging, or atherosclerosis.

Anticonvulsive

As a nervine and sedative Clary Sage is also an anticonvulsive, which means it helps relieve and reduce convulsive fits, whether epileptic or induced by another form of nervous or psychological condition.

Common Therapeutic Uses

Traditionally used to enhance the body's defenses against women's issues, Clary Sage essential oil remains a significant support for feminine wellness; protecting against a number of conditions that affect women. Clary Sage supports menstrual and menopausal wellness, while mentally uplifting and reducing blood pressure. Let's take a closer look at the common uses for this oil.

Women's Wellness

Clary Sage can significantly benefit women at any age, as it helps balance hormones. Female hormones fluctuate significantly, resulting in the fluctuation of bodily function and the psyche. In some cases, this hormonal imbalance can impact their daily lives. This is why administering Clary Sage, particularly during periods of menstrual or menopausal influx, can support the body's natural function. If you commonly experience painful, irregular periods, or unpleasant menopausal effects, a Clary Sage application will help relieve menstrual- or menopausal-related condition. The oil can help young women become regular and relieve painful menstrual cramps, while helping aging women combat unpleasant attributes of menopause, like hot flashes and mood-swings, all by better maintaining hormonal balance. Clary Sage essential oil also helps regulate other gynecological conditions, protecting against uterine cancer by regulating estrogen production, thereby decreasing the risk of uterine cyst and tumor formation after menopause.

Skin Tone & Condition

Clary Sage contains an ester called linalyl acetate. This ester helps heal rashes and other skin imperfections, as it serves skin as an anti-inflammatory. It also supports all skin types – oily or dry – by maintaining and balancing oil production in the skin. As a topical antiseptic, Clary Sage also supports your body's defenses against infections in wounds, as well as in burns and blisters. Moreover, Clary Sage is an antifungal and so can help protect against fungal infections, which can be highly contagious.

Boosts Libido

The slightly nutty fragrance of Clary Sage relaxes the body and at the same time, makes one feel euphoric. The result is a sensual essential oil that is both an aphrodisiac, a hormone balancer, and libido stimulant for men and women. This oil may also aid in cases of erectile dysfunction and infertility.

Helps Reduce Blood Pressure

As a hypotensive, Clary Sage effectively reduces blood pressure by supporting the relaxation of veins and arteries, Clary Sage effectively reduces blood pressure. This supports overall wellness, as everything in the body – your blood vessels, brain, muscles, and other organs – functions better with increased circulation and oxygenation. Your risks for such issues as stroke, heart attack, brain hemorrhaging, or atherosclerosis are reduced and even your metabolism is given a jolt when blood pressure is optimal.

Stomach Wellness

Clary Sage is a digestive, a carminative, an antispasmodic, and an emmenagogue and therefore is an effective support when it comes to stomach wellness. Whether you have menstrual cramps, indigestion, nausea, or upset stomach, a dosage of this oil and its supportive properties will help ease the pain and uncomfortable nature of most any stomach issue, while maintaining overall wellness of the gastrointestinal tract.

Supports Depression

The scent of Clary Sage has been shown to relieve anxiety and depression, soothing emotion and calming nerves. The oil is both a euphoric and a natural sedative, meaning that it uplifts the spirit, while easing mental fatigue, nervousness, and exhaustion. If you are feeling stressed, you can combat your negative emotions or head them off through a Clary Sage essential oil application, whether aroma-therapeutic, ingested, or topical.

Safety Precautions & Common Applications

Safety

Certain adverse effects may evolve when using pure essential oils. Some essential oils should not be used when pregnant, for example, as they may cause miscarriage. Allergic reactions may occur especially when applied topically. Always administer an allergy test before committing fully to topical application. When used with other medications essential oils may react negatively. If you are on any current prescription medications or have a chronic illness, such as high blood pressure, epilepsy or liver disease, then researching the effects of essential oils against your own personal medical history will eliminate any potentially problematic issues.

Clary Sage has been approved by the FDA for internal consumption and so can be used as a dietary supplement. Do not use when drinking alcohol, as Clary Sage has a narcotic effect. Those who have breast cancer should avoid Clary Sage, as it also has an estrogen-like effect. If you have sensitive skin, dilute heavily and test before extensive use. Otherwise, dilute 1:1 with a carrier oil. You can apply topically, diffuse or use as a dietary supplement.

Blends

Oftentimes essential oils are manufactured as blends of several pure oils. For instance, the Protective Blend of certain brands is a mix of cinnamon, clove, rosemary, and eucalyptus. This blend can be used to boost the immune system to help support colds, viruses and flus. The downside to blends is that the more oils added to the mix, the higher the probability your patient may react negatively to the blend if he/she is prone to allergies. There is also the possibility of phototoxicity when working with blends, particularly if they include citrus oils. Be sure to read your labels before administering.

Regardless of these possible effects, essential oils are a viable option for supporting a number of conditions. Those looking to support or maintain their own personal wellness, or that of their families', should become educated on the uses of essential oils, their natural remedies and the methods of application. Only then can you begin building your kit of essential oils for survival

Chapter 2:
Recipes for Clary Sage Essential Oil

In this chapter, we will offer various recipes for Clary Sage essential oil, both for pure Clary Sage applications and blends. For pure applications, we have provided the appropriate application and dosage to support specific ailments, from addiction to viral infections. When it comes to blends, herbalists, and aromatherapists often combine Clary Sage essential oil with sandalwood, frankincense, lavender, juniper, pine, jasmine, juniper, lemon, lime, orange and other citrus fruits. We will offer some fantastic blending options in the second half of this chapter.

Pure Applications

Amenorrhea

Amenorrhea, or skipping a menstrual cycle, can be avoided by diluting Clary Sage essential oil in a 1:1 ratio with a carrier oil and applying topically over the lower abdomen, as well as into the ankles and the soles of the feet.

Aneurysm

To protect against aneurysm, dilute Clary Sage essential oil in a 1:1 ratio with a carrier oil and apply topically, massaging over the heart and into the reflex points of the feet on a daily basis. For added support diffuse throughout the room.

Aphrodisiac

Clary Sage has long been used to stimulate the libido. Diffuse regularly or dilute Clary Sage essential oil with a carrier oil and apply topically to the soles of the feet.

Cholesterol Levels

Promote healthy cholesterol levels by diluting Clary Sage essential oil in a 1:1 ratio with a carrier oil and massaging over the heart and into the reflex points of the feet.

Courage

To enhance confidence, place a drop of Clary Sage essential oil into your hands, rub your palms together, cup them over your nose, and breathe deeply in and out for several minutes. Use daily for the best results.

Confusion

Relieve confusion by applying a single drop of Clary Sage across the brow.

Convulsions

Eliminate convulsions by supporting your body's balance and calming the nervous system. Dilute Clary Sage essential oil in a 1:1 ratio with a carrier oil and massage into the reflex points of the feet and into the neck three times daily.

Cramps

Alleviate menstrual, intestinal, or abdominal cramps by diluting Clary Sage essential oil in a 1:1 ratio with a carrier oil and applying topically. Massage into the lower abdomen and back and into the reflex points of the feet.

Creativity

Clary Sage can serve as a stimulant for creativity. Apply a single drop over the brow every 1-4 hours as needed.

Depression

Combat depression by directly inhaling or by placing a

drop of Clary Sage essential oil on your pillow, in your water or tea. You can also diffuse throughout the room or dilute the oil in a 1:1 ratio with a carrier oil and apply topically, massaging into scalp, neck and shoulders.

Digestive Aid

Clary Sage supports the digestive tract. Dilute the oil in a 1:1 ratio with a carrier oil and apply topically to the abdomen in a clockwise motion and into the reflex points of the feet. You can also diffuse throughout the home.

Doubt

If you are experiencing self-doubt, pour a drop of Clary Sage essential oil into your hands, rub your palms together, cup them over your nose, and breathe deeply in and out for several minutes. Apply topically to the brow or throat.

Dysmenorrhea

Dysmenorrhea, or painful periods, can be avoided by diluting Clary Sage essential oil in a 1:1 ratio with a carrier oil and applying topically over the lower abdomen, as well as into the ankles and the arches of the feet.

Endometriosis

To combat endometriosis, dilute Clary Sage essential oil in a 1:1 ratio with a carrier oil and massage into the lower back and into the reflex points of the feet three times daily.

Epilepsy

Support epilepsy by applying a drop of Clary Sage to the brow or base of the neck twice daily.

Estrogen Enhancer

Clary Sage can function as a phytoestrogen, which aids the body's cells in the production of estrogen. To administer dilute Clary Sage essential oil in a 1:1 ratio with a carrier oil and massage into the reflex points of the feet and into the lower abdomen over the ovaries once a day.

Frigidity

If you are experiencing frigidity, pour a drop of Clary Sage essential oil into your hands, rub your palms together, cup them over your nose, and breathe deeply in and out for several minutes.

Hair (Fragile)

For fragile hair, dilute Clary Sage essential oil in a 1:1 ratio with a carrier oil and massage into the reflex points of the feet once daily.

Hopelessness

If you are feeling dejected or hopeless, inhale deeply and directly when needed.

Hormonal Balance

Support hormonal balance by diluting Clary Sage essential oil in a 1:1 ratio with a carrier oil and massaging into the reflex points of the feet daily.

Hot Flashes

Clary Sage is ideal for hot flashes. To apply, dilute Clary Sage essential oil in a 1:1 ratio with a carrier oil and massage into the back of the neck daily or whenever a hot flash occurs. Place a few drops in a spray bottle full of distilled water and spritz it over the body for fast-acting relief.

Impotency Support

Clary Sage enhances circulation and relaxes the muscles. The oil is also said to aid in issues of impotency and also support fertility. To administer, dilute Clary Sage essential oil in a 1:1 ratio with a carrier oil and massage into the reflex points of the feet.

Infection

To fight off infection, dilute Clary Sage essential oil in a 1:1 ratio with a carrier oil and apply topically to the affected area or to the soles of the feet. You can also diffuse throughout the room; whichever application is more appropriate to your specific infection.

Infertility

Stimulate fertility by diluting Clary Sage essential oil in a 1:1 ratio with a carrier oil and apply topically, massaging over the reproductive organs and into the reflex points of the feet. You can also diffuse throughout the room for a similar effect.

Insomnia

With its calming and relaxing scent, Clary Sage essential oil can help fight insomnia. Dilute Clary Sage essential oil in a 1:1 ratio with a carrier oil and massage into the reflex points of the feet and into the back of the neck to trigger nervous system response. You might also diffuse or place a couple drops on your pillow or sheets.

Lactation (Increasing)

Increase lactation by diluting Clary Sage essential oil in a 1:1 ratio with a carrier oil and apply topically, massaging into the breasts toward the lymph nodes (underarms) twice daily.

Menopause

Support the body's natural defenses against menopausal symptoms by applying Clary Sage essential oil topically over the chest, lower abdomen, and into the soles of the feet. You can also diffuse throughout the home to maintain hormonal balance.

Mood Swings

Maintain mood balance by diffusing Clary Sage essential oil throughout the home. If making concentrated efforts to stave off mood swings, inhale directly for 30 seconds or more throughout the day or dilute Clary Sage essential oil in a 1:1 ratio with a carrier oil and massage into the reflex points of the feet.

Muscle Fatigue

To relieve muscle fatigue, dilute Clary Sage essential oil in a 1:1 ratio with a carrier oil and massage the solution into the affected area, toward the heart.

Parkinson's Disease

Support the symptoms of Parkinson's Disease by diluting Clary Sage essential oil in a 1:1 ratio with a carrier oil and massaging into the back of the neck and into the reflex points of the feet.

PMS

Relieve PMS symptoms by diffusing throughout your cycle. You can also dilute Clary Sage essential oil in a 1:1 ratio with a carrier oil and massage it into the reflex points of the feet on a regular basis throughout the month.

Postpartum Depression

To relieve postpartum depression, diffuse Clary Sage essential oil throughout the home. You can also inhale directly, put a drop on your shirt collar, or place a drop in your palms, rub your hands together, and run them through your hair. To further support depression, dilute Clary Sage essential oil in a 1:1 ratio with a carrier oil and massage into the reflex points of the feet.

Seizures

Protect against or relieve seizures by diluting Clary Sage essential oil in a 1:1 ratio with a carrier oil and massaging into the chest, back of the neck, and into the reflex points of the feet. This will calm the body's nervous system.

Skin (Dry, Sensitive, Eczema, Psoriasis, etc)

Clary Sage can be used for all sorts of skin conditions. Apply Clary Sage essential oil directly to the affected area or, for sensitive skin, dilute with your daily skin care regimen.

Stress

Combat stress by steaming two drops of Clary Sage essential oil in a pan of water, remove the steaming pan from the stove, pour into a bowl, place a towel over your head and inhale. You can also diffuse throughout the room or place a drop onto your shirt collar for portable stress relief.

Blends

Appetite Stimulant

Ingredients

8 drops Clary Sage Essential Oil

6 drops Coriander Essential Oil

4 drops Black Pepper Essential oil

3 drops Ginger Essential Oil

2 drops Peppermint Essential Oil

Directions

To help stimulate appetite, diffuse throughout the home or pour the blend into your inhalant to use throughout the day. Those who have recently been ill or going through chemotherapy can boost their appetite through frequent inhalation.

Creative Stimulant

Ingredients

1 drop Lime Essential Oil

1 drop Clary Sage Essential Oil

1 drop Sandalwood Essential Oil

3 drops Carrier Oil

Directions

To stimulate creativity, combine ingredients in a small glass container and apply topically to your pulse points.

De-stress Bath

Ingredients

2 drops Rosemary Essential Oil

3 drops Black Pepper Essential Oil

5 drops Grapefruit Essential Oil

1 Tbsp Grapeseed Oil

Directions

To wind down, de-stress, and combat anxiety, add all ingredients to your bathwater and stir to disperse. Then inhale deeply while you soak for 20 minutes, but avoid getting water in your eyes, as it may sting.

Fallen Arches

Ingredients

5 drops Black Pepper Essential Oil

5 drops Clary Sage Essential Oil

10 drops Ginger Essential Oil

10 drops Rosemary Essential Oil

2 Tsp Carrier Oil

Directions

To relieve the stress of fallen arches, combine all ingredients in a small bowl, blending well. Apply to the instep of the foot, massaging toward the heel.

Fatigue

Ingredients

1 drops Ginger Essential Oil

2 drops Clary Sage Essential Oil

2 drops Sandalwood Essential Oil

2 drops Cilantro Essential Oil

3 drops Frankincense Essential Oil

½ Tbsp Carrier Oil

Directions

To combat fatigue, combine all ingredients in a small bowl or container, blending well. Apply topically to the forearms and the back of the neck, inhaling the scent deeply.

Fingernails/Cuticles

Ingredients

3 drops Lemon Essential Oil

3 drops Geranium Essential Oil

3 drops Rosemary Essential Oil

6 drops Clary Sage Essential Oil

6 drops Lavender Essential Oil

1 ounce Jojoba Oil

1 ounce Sweet Almond Oil

Directions

To promote healthy nails and cuticles, especially after
exposing your hands to harsh chemicals, combine all
ingredients in a small bowl, blending well. Before you
go to bed, apply a single drop topically to each nail and
cuticle, massaging over the nail.

Hot Flash Relief

Ingredients

2 drops Peppermint Essential Oil

2 drops Clary Sage Essential Oil

4 drops Geranium Essential Oil

4 drops Bergamot Essential Oil

10 drops Lavender Essential Oil

8 ounces Witch Hazel (alcohol free)

Directions

To help relieve hot flashes, combine all ingredients in a glass spray bottle and use as needed. Shake vigorously before each use.

Hot Flash Relief II

Ingredients

1 drop Fennel Essential Oil

1 drop Palmarosa Essential Oil

1 drop Clary Sage Essential Oil

3 drops Carrier Oil

Directions

Relieve hot flashes by combining all ingredients in a small glass container and applying topically to your pulse points.

Insomnia

Ingredients

1 drop Clary Sage Essential Oil

3 drops Lavender Essential Oil

1 tsp Cream

Directions

To relieve insomnia, fill the tub with warm water and pour in the essential oils, stirring the tub until evenly distributed. Soak in the bath for 15-20 minutes.

Joyful Blend

Ingredients

1 drop Lavender Essential Oil

1 drop Clary Sage Essential Oil

1 drop Roman Chamomile Essential Oil

1 drop Geranium Essential Oil

Directions

To promote joy and euphoria, diffuse this blend throughout your home.

Joyful Mist

Ingredients

10 drops Frankincense Essential Oil

8 drops Orange Essential Oil

7 drops Clary Sage Essential Oil

48 mL Distilled Water

1 mL Vodka

Directions

For a joyful mist spray, combine ingredients in a 50mL glass spray bottle and spray throughout your room, study, or vehicle at the end of a tough day. Shake well before each use.

Menstrual Cramps

Ingredients

3 drops Basil Essential Oil

3 drops Clary Sage Essential Oil

3 drops Coconut Oil

Directions

To relieve menstrual cramps, place all ingredients into a small bowl or container and blend thoroughly then administer topically, massaging into the abdomen every hour until pain is eliminated. Drink water for added support.

No Limits Spray

Ingredients

12 drops Mandarin Essential Oil

6 drops Geranium Essential Oil

6 drops Clary Sage Essential Oil

3 drops Cinnamon Essential Oil

48 mL Distilled Water

1 mL Vodka

Directions

For a confidence boosting mist spray that leaves you limitless, combine ingredients in a 50mL glass spray bottle and spray throughout your room, study, or vehicle when needed. Shake well before each use.

Ovarian Cyst

Ingredients

2 drops Thyme Essential Oil

2 drops Rosemary Essential Oil

5 drops Clary Sage Essential Oil

5 drops Myrrh Essential Oil

9 drops Frankincense Essential Oil

Directions

In a small bowl or container, mix all ingredients until well combined. Apply 1-3 drops on the respective reflex points on the anklebones on either side of the feet. You can also apply with a warm compress over the area of concern.

PMS

Ingredients

5 drops Clary Sage Essential Oil

5 drops Rose Essential Oil

3 drops Bergamot Essential Oil

2 ounces Jojoba Oil

Directions

In a small bowl or container, mix all ingredients until well combined. To help relax, relieve sore muscles, and promote healthy emotion, apply in a full-body massage.

Stress Relief

Ingredients

25 drops Wild Orange Essential Oil

20 drops Grapefruit Essential Oil

15 drops Frankincense Essential Oil

15 drops Bergamot Essential Oil

10 drops Clary Sage Essential Oil

10 drops Lemon Essential Oil

Directions

To help focus concentration, diffuse throughout the home or office.

Stress Relief II

Ingredients

1 drop Marjoram Essential Oil

1 drop Lavender Essential Oil

1 drop Clary Sage Essential Oil

3 drops Carrier Oil

Directions

Relieve stress by combining all ingredients in a small glass container and applying topically to your pulse points.

Chapter 3:
Clary Sage Essential Oil Studies

Many studies have been done on essential oils to uncover and prove their therapeutic qualities. In the case of the great number of Clary Sage studies, many of the properties attributed to the essential oil (noted in this book and elsewhere) are quite often validated through the research from accredited universities and published by reputable scientific journals. In this chapter, we will discuss a small portion of these studies. It is important to note that research on essential oils is constant and evolving. Keep up with any recent research as it may turn up even further valuable uses of these miracle oils.

Study 1 – Urinary Incontinence

In this study available on PubMed, the analgesic effects of Clary Sage essential oil on the autonomic nervous system were examined, with the following results: "The aim of this study was to investigate the effect of inhalation of Salvia sclarea (Clary Sage) essential oil vapors on autonomic nervous system activity in female patients with urinary incontinence undergoing urodynamic assessment. These results suggest that clary oil inhalation may be useful in inducing relaxation in female urinary incontinence patients undergoing urodynamic assessments."

Urinary incontinence is involuntary urination or leakage of urine, which can be distressing and can significantly affect an individual's quality of life. This study analyzed the effects of lavender and Clary Sage essential oil vapors on the autonomic nervous system activity in women that influences urinary incontinence.

The double-blind, randomized, controlled study involved 34 patients who suffer from the condition. The women were divided into three groups, which included the 60-minute inhalation of either Clary Sage, lavender, and almond (the control group). Pre- and post-measurements of the patients' blood pressure, respiratory and pulse rates, and salivary cortisol were taken. Clary Sage had the best results when it came to decreasing blood pressure and respiratory rate, which indicates that the inhalation of Clary Sage essential oil may support those suffering from urinary incontinence.

Reference:
http://www.ncbi.nlm.nih.gov/pubmed/23360656]

http://www.ncbi.nlm.nih.gov/pmc/articles/PMC3700459/
pdf/acm.2012.0148.pdf]

Study 2 – Menstruation (Dysmenorrhea)

In this study available on PubMed, the effects of an essential oil blend containing Clary Sage on menstruation were examined, with the following results: "This study assessed the effectiveness of blended essential oils on menstrual cramps for outpatients with primary dysmenorrhea and explored the analgesic ingredients in the essential oils…Essential oils blended with lavender (Lavandula officinalis), Clary Sage (Salvia sclarea) and marjoram (Origanum majorana) in a 2:1:1 ratio was diluted in unscented cream at 3% concentration for the essential oil group…The duration of pain was significantly reduced from 2.4 to 1.8 days after aromatherapy intervention in the essential oil group. Aromatic oil massage provided relief for outpatients with primary dysmenorrhea and reduced the duration of menstrual pain in the essential oil group. This study suggests that this blended formula can serve as a reference for alternative and complementary medicine on primary dysmenorrhea."

This study demonstrated the efficacy of an essential oil blend – consisting of lavender, Clary Sage, and marjoram diluted in cream – against excessive menstrual bleeding and pain, a condition known as dysmenorrhea. After massaging the essential oil into the abdominal area daily from the final day of one menstruation period to the first day of the next, both the amount of bleeding and pain were significantly reduced. The study attributes this result to the combined effects of the analgesic components in the oils: linalyl acetate, linalool, eucalyptol, and β-caryophyllene.

Reference:
http://www.ncbi.nlm.nih.gov/pubmed/22435409]

Study 3 – Antidepressant Properties

In this study available on PubMed, the antidepressant effects of Clary Sage essential oil were examined, with the following results: "The purpose of this study was to examine the antidepressant-like effects of Clary Sage oil on human beings by comparing the neurotransmitter level change in plasma...[the results indicate that] Clary Sage oil has antidepressant-like effect, and KBDI-II inventory may be the most sensitive and valid tool in screening for depression status or severity."

This study analyzed the effects of Clary Sage essential oil on depression in menopausal women. 22 women over

50 years of age participated, divided into two groups: a normal- or depressed-tendency group. The study showed that following the inhalation of Clary Sage essential oil, 5-hydroxytryptamine (5-HT) concentration was significantly increased, while cortisol levels were reduced. 5-hydroxytryptamine is commonly known as serotonin, and is believed to contribute to feelings of happiness and overall well-being. Cortisol is released in response to stress. These results suggest that Clary Sage can be effectively used as an antidepressant.

Reference:
http://www.ncbi.nlm.nih.gov/pubmed/24802524]

Study 4 – Antidepressant Properties

In this study available on PubMed, the antidepressant effects of Clary Sage essential oil were examined, with the following results: "The purpose of the present study was to screen aromatic essential oils that have antidepressant effects to identify the regulatory mechanisms of selected essential oils…Our findings indicate that clary oil could be developed as a therapeutic agent for patients with depression and that the antidepressant-like effect of clary oil is closely associated with modulation of the DAnergic pathway."

This study was a comparative analysis of the effects of several essential oils – including rosemary, chamomile, lavender, and Clary Sage – on stress and depression, measured by pre- and post-test statistics on rats before and after a forced swim test.

Clary Sage was discovered to have the strongest anti-stressor effect. The oil's antidepressant properties were further tested by pretreatment with antagonists to adrenaline, serotonin, dopamine, and GABA receptors. The results were positive across the board, indicating that Clary Sage essential oil may effectively support depression and like conditions.

Reference & Photo Credit:
http://www.ncbi.nlm.nih.gov/pubmed/20441789]

Study 5 – Childbirth

In this study available on PubMed, the effects of Clary Sage essential oil on childbirth were examined, with the following results: "The authors report the process and results of an evaluation of a midwifery aromatherapy service for mothers in labor…a key finding of this study suggests that two essential oils, Clary Sage and chamomile are effective in alleviating pain. The evidence from this study suggests that aromatherapy can be effective in reducing maternal anxiety, fear and/or pain during labor. The use of aromatherapy appeared to facilitate a further reduction in the use of systemic opioids in the study center, from 6% in 1990 to 0.4% in 1997 (per woman).

Aromatherapy is an inexpensive care option…The successful model of integrated practice that this aromatherapy study presents, offers a useful example for other units to consider."

Taking place over an 8-year period, this study is the most expansive research initiative when it comes to applying aromatherapy in a healthcare setting. The study took a look at 8058 mothers in childbirth, with a wide ranging group that included spontaneous labor and birth, induced labor, Caesarean section, and vaginal operative delivery. Ten essential oils were tested, through skin absorption and inhalation therapy. Clary Sage was amongst the two essential oils that effectively alleviated pain during labor.

Reference & Photo Credit:
http://www.ncbi.nlm.nih.gov/pubmed/11033651]

Study 6 – Repellency

In this study published by the *Journal of Anthropod-Borne Diseases*, the repellent effects of Clary Sage essential oil were examined, with the following results: "Using special lotions and repellent sprays on skin is one of the effective methods to prevent Arthropods biting which was verified in this study…Essential oils of Salvia sclarea, Lavendula officinalis and Myrtus communis have repellency effect, even with

10% concentration of essential oils."

This was a controlled study in which WHO guidelines for efficacy testing of mosquito repellents for human skin were applied to various concentrations of the solutions applied to positive and negative control groups. The positive controls included traditional repellents (DEET) and the negative controls were naked hands and those sprayed with ethanol. Four plant essential oils were tested, including Clary Sage.

Pre- and post-study measurements were recorded, including the number and rate of bug bites, according to each concentration. The results indicate that Clary Sage essential oil can effectively repel mosquitos, even at a 10% concentration.

Reference:
http://www.ncbi.nlm.nih.gov/pubmed/25629066]

http://www.ncbi.nlm.nih.gov/pmc/articles/PMC4289512/pdf/jad-8-60.pdf]

Chapter 4:
The Ins & Outs of Essential Oils

Where do essential oils come from?

Plants and plant species naturally produce essential oils for various reasons, one being to draw pollinator insects to them, another being to repel invading organisms (bacteria, animals). A number of chemical compounds compose each plant's essential oil, and the combination of these compounds are specific to each oil, which then instills in the oil its own unique properties. Essential oils can be harnessed from all sorts of plant components, including flowers, leaves, bark, fruit, roots, and resin. For instance, cinnamon oil is harnessed from bark, lemon oil from the peel, and lavender oil from flowers. Certain plants can produce a few chemical variants of the same essential oil, which are acquired from different parts of the plant. Some of these parts produce a large amount of oil, while others produce just a smidgen. The oil's quality and potency depends upon a number of factors, including the subspecies of the plant, its soil conditions, the time of year, and even the time of day you harvest it.

How are essential oils extracted?

Essential oils can be extracted from plants through various methods, including pressing, distillation, solvent, and maceration. Let's take a brief look at each:

Pressing Method

Commonly used with citrus fruit, the pressing method extracts the oil through a technique which involves pushing the fruit peels through a press. Oily fruits and plants are best suited for this technique. Orange oil, for example, is extracted from orange skins through the pressing method.

Distillation Method

This technique harkens back to the days of moonshiners, as the same sort of method used to create strong liquor can be used to extract essential oils. Using a still, boiled water, and plant materials, will create steam which is then cooled by coils and condensed into a combination of water and oil. This combination does not mix, so the oil can then be extracted from it.

Solvent Method

Through a multi-step process, certain plant and flower oils can be extracted using alcohol and other solvents, which extract the essential oils from the plant materials.

Maceration Method

When a "carrier," fixed oil, or lard is mixed with the plant material and set out in the sun over a period of time, the carrier oil is infused with the plant's essence. Heat sources, other than the sun, are often used to speed the process. Throughout the process more plant material is added to produce a more potent oil.

How do you use essential oils?

Although some studies about the effectiveness of essential oils are conducted by small companies, or even individuals, a number of them are conducted by the food and cosmetic industries. In general, the pharmaceutical industry shows next to no interest in herbal medicine, primarily because there are few options to patent such products. As such, the product's lack of profitability results in a lack of research funding. Regardless, the historical uses of essential oils tell us what we need to know; these oils have been effectively administered for centuries. The therapeutic qualifications of essential oils can be plotted in the survival of the human race across cultures and generations.

Another reason that studies on essential oils have not

resulted in much conclusive evidence as to their overall effectiveness is because definitive results are sometimes difficult to prove, as the quality of each batch of oil can vary for a number of reasons. One is that essential oils are impossible to standardize. As mentioned above, even the slightest variance in soil conditions, and the time of harvesting – as well as innumerable other factors – will produce a different product quality and potency. In addition, essential oils are often obtained from various species of the same plant; Eucalyptus radiata and Eucalyptus globulus can both be used in the making of therapeutic-grade eucalyptus oil, as a result, they may have slightly different properties and degrees of strength or effectiveness.

Just as there are a number of methods by which to extract essential oils, there are a number of methods to administer them therapeutically. The variety of chemical compounds in each essential oil means that their benefits and applications also vary across the board. Below are a few of these methods.

Topical Administration

Direct application of many essential oils works like a sponge, as skin absorbs chemicals and other things (like sunlight, for instance). Topical application is best for clearing up an ailment on the skin's surface, or in the underlying muscle tissue. When applying topically, massage the oil into the skin, or simply dab on the skin for therapeutic results. Combine the essential oil with a carrier oil for topical use in order to dilute its potency. This is safer as the oil is concentrated. Support the body's defenses against rash or muscle pain in this manner, but always test the patient for allergens before applying. Adverse effects are produced by natural chemicals as much as synthetic ones; poison ivy, for example.

To test for allergens, place a drop or two on the patient's inner forearm. If a rash develops within 12 to 24 hours, then the patient is allergic. In addition, phototoxicity – sun exposure resulting in an exacerbated burn – may be an issue when citrus oils are applied topically. One must proceed with caution when applying essential oils using this method.

Inhalation Therapy

Commonly known as "aromatherapy," this essential oil application is effective for inner ailments, like sore throat, or cold. In a steaming bowl of distilled, or sterilized water, add a few drops of essential oil, then with a towel over your head, bend over the bowl and inhale. The towel captures the vapors, making the technique even more effective. Essential oils can also be placed in a diffuser, or potpourri throughout a room, to produce somewhat diluted therapeutic effects.

Ingestion

When using this method, proceed with caution. Direct ingestion of essential oils must be monitored and applied in small doses that are diluted in a tablespoon or more of any carrier oil – olive oil, for example. If you are unsure of dosage amounts, make a tea with the relevant herb instead. Although the effects of this diluted use may be weaker, this application is a better alternative than an overdose of essential oils.

What are the general benefits of using essential oils?

Supplement for Prescription Drugs

One practical benefit of using essential oils is their supplemental nature; which is the ultimate reason to learn about their administration, and begin stockpiling an essential oil supply. One of the potential threats of economic/social collapse is the lack of resources, and primarily the inability to procure prescription drugs. As such, finding suitable alternatives should be a priority when prepping for the worst.

Their portability is also a major bonus when it comes to survival prepping. The fact that these ultra-concentrated oils take up little-to-no space makes toting them all the simpler should the need arise. Because essential oils are highly concentrated, the application used in most methods of administration requires only a drop or two of oil, which means that tiny bottle will last a long time.

Cost Effective Supplement

Though money may be the last thing on your mind when it comes to prepping for a survival situation (money may even be obsolete in the event of social collapse), it is worth noting that the expense of essential oils pales in comparison to prescription drugs. Essential oils are an inexpensive, effective supplement to prescription medicine.

No Expiration Date

Another benefit of essential oils is that they do not expire, nor do they have "proper storage" requirements. A number of medicines, and medicinal products, must be replaced every few years; this sets essential oils ahead of the pack when it comes to shelf life.

Versatility

Essential oils also offer great versatility. Aside from providing wellness benefits, essential oils can be repurposed for household and hygienic applications. For instance, if looking for something that might serve dental hygiene needs in a time of crisis, then thieves oil is a go-to essential oil. To maintain the skin's tone and condition, frankincense and lavender will do the trick; the latter also serves as sunscreen, preventing sun damage as well.

When it comes to the house or shelter, use essential oils to deodorize, which will come in handy in a disaster scenario, especially if things start to smell due to lack of proper utilities and maintenance. For example, after the 2011 tsunami and the subsequent nuclear reactor meltdown in Japan, a nurse named Risa Nakahira used essential oils to deodorize and sanitize putrid public bathrooms in overpopulated evacuation facilities. As relief workers searched for survivors, often wading through debris and decay, Nakahira also deodorized their boots and masks using essential oils. The possibilities of these natural oils are endless.

They are also versatile when it comes to the range of patients they are capable of supporting. The wellness of everyone, from a great grandfather to an infant baby, can be fortified with the aid of essential oils in the appropriate dosage. They even come in handy when treating livestock or pets. From teething infants to dementia in the elderly, from teenagers with acne to dogs with urinary tract infections, essential oils can serve any patient with nearly any ailment.

Conclusion

Now that you know all about what Clary Sage essential oil can do for you – where it originates, how it is extracted, the benefits and properties, and the different methods of administration – use it confidently to support the body's defenses against wellness issues and start to assemble a kit of essential oils for survival. Essential oils can be purchased online or at your local holistic treatment store.

The various benefits of essential oils and their properties are countless. To build a kit, first focus on acquiring the essential oils which may bear more relevance to personal wellness issues, or the potential health threats, within the environment. In the event of a viral outbreak, for instance, Clary Sage essential oil will be one of the more crucial oils – along with oregano, lemon, frankincense, and cinnamon (eBooks also available for purchase) – due to their antiviral and immuno-supportive properties.

Used as a supplement or as the go-to for skin conditions, infections, or immune-boosting agents, the application of Clary Sage essential oil in medicine has survived for centuries and will survive centuries more. When it comes down to it, we do not need to rely on pharmaceuticals; essential oils, herbs, and plenty of other natural ingredients can be used to help support the body's natural defenses against any number of wellness issues; ailment or injury.

Essential oils are essential to your survival in the case of viral outbreak, social collapse, or natural disaster because, when the SHTF, access to pharmaceuticals will likely be limited, or obsolete altogether. Alternatives to our modern-day standard will equate survival when no other option exists

DISCLAIMER AND/OR LEGAL NOTICES: Every effort has been made to accurately represent this book and it's potential. Results vary with every individual, and your results may or may not be different from those depicted. No promises, guarantees or warranties, whether stated or implied, have been made that you will produce any specific result from this book. Your efforts are individual and unique, and may vary from those shown. Your success depends on your efforts, background and motivation.

The material in this publication is provided for educational and informational purposes only and is not intended as medical advice. The information contained in this book should not be used to diagnose or treat any illness, metabolic disorder, disease or health problem. Always consult your physician or healthcare provider before beginning any nutrition or exercise program. Use of the programs, advice, and information contained in this book is at the sole choice and risk of the reader.

www.ingramcontent.com/pod-product-compliance
Lightning Source LLC
Chambersburg PA
CBHW062109280526
45788CB00003B/1407